TABLE OF CONTENTS

DISCLAIMER AND TERMS OF USE AGREEMENT.

Introduction

Chapter 1 – The Andropause Mystery

Chapter 2 - Beat Male Menopause - Testosterone Replacement Therapy

Chapter 3 - A Guide in Surviving Male Menopause for Men and Women

Chapter 4 - Male Menopaws: The Silent Howl

Chapter 5 - Mr. Hyde and Dr. Jekyll Syndrome vs. Male Menopause

Chapter 6 - Male Menopause Phase

Chapter 7 - Male Menopause and Depression

Chapter 8 - Testosterone Talk: Symptoms of Male Menopause

Chapter 9 - What You Must Do To Treat Male Menopause

I Have a Special Gift for My Readers

Meet the Author

How To Cope with Male Menopause
The Andropause Mystery Revealed
©Copyright 2013 by Dr. Treat Preston

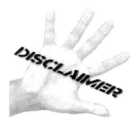

DISCLAIMER AND TERMS OF USE AGREEMENT:

(Please Read This Before Using This Book)

This information is for educational and informational purposes only. The content is not intended to be a substitute for any professional advice, diagnosis, or treatment.

The authors and publisher of this book and the accompanying materials have used their best efforts in preparing this book.

The authors and publisher make no representation or warranties with respect to the accuracy, applicability, fitness, or completeness of the contents of this book. The information contained in this book is strictly for educational purposes. Therefore, if you wish to apply ideas contained in this book, you are taking full responsibility for your actions.

The authors and publisher disclaim any warranties (express or implied), merchantability, or fitness for any particular purpose. The author and publisher shall in no event be held liable to any party for any direct, indirect, punitive, special, incidental or other consequential damages arising directly or indirectly from any use of this material, which is provided "as is", and without warranties. As always, the advice of a competent legal, tax, accounting, medical or other professional should be sought where applicable.

The authors and publisher do not warrant the performance, effectiveness or applicability of any sites listed or linked to in this book. All links are for information purposes only and are not warranted for content, accuracy or any other implied or explicit purpose. No part of this may be copied, or changed in any format, or used in any way other than what is outlined within this course under any circumstances. Violators will be prosecuted.

This book is © Copyrighted by ePubWealth.com.

Introduction

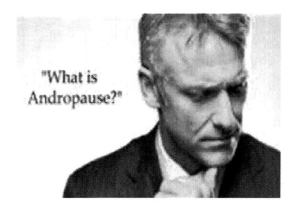

How To Cope with Male Menopause - The Andropause Mystery Revealed is all about the controversial subject of male menopause or "andropause". It discusses in detail what male menopause is, male menopause symptoms, male menopause treatment, andropause, HRT or hormone replacement therapy, and hormone imbalance.

Women may not be the only ones who suffer the effects of changing hormones. Some doctors are noticing that men are reporting some of the same symptoms that women experience in perimenopause and menopause.

The medical community is debating whether or not men really do go through a well-defined menopause. Doctors say that men receiving hormone therapy with testosterone have reported relief of some of the symptoms associated with so-called male menopause. Because men do not go through a well-defined period referred to as menopause, some doctors refer to this problem as androgen (testosterone) decline in the aging male -- or what some people call low testosterone.

Men do experience a decline in the production of the male hormone testosterone with aging, but this also occurs with conditions such as diabetes.

In this book, I want to get into a detailed discussion of male menopause so that my readers can see if they fit into the descriptions provided herein and then seek proper medical attention.

Chapter 1 – The Andropause Mystery

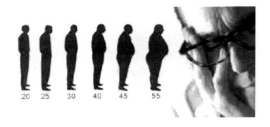

When a man enters the age of forty, he begins to experience the awkward feeling of confusion, split personality and stressfulness. He tends to lose his sense of purpose as well as his former self. He is craving for the new order of things, more ventures and is spinning out of control.

In the quest to understand this crisis, series of studies are undertaken. Even the medical science allots time to formulate possible formulas to find the remedy on its symptoms. There are creams, pellets, pills and even surgeries that are deemed to resolve the crisis.

But what is really in the core of this predicament? Dr. Robert S. Tan constructed his book of Andropause mystery: unraveling the truths about male menopause in the pursuit to explain the circumstances and why they happen to a man.

According to Dr. Robert Tan, menopause or the declination of hormonal levels comes to pass to both men and women. For men, such transition period is called andropause. The period usually strikes at forty when age normally causes internal troubles to almost everyone.

Subsequently, internal changes had exterior manifestations in terms of social, career and family interactions.

Furthermore, Dr. Robert Tan added that as the man reaches the age of 50-70, the symptoms become more visible and provoked. Symptoms such as declination of levels of virility and energy accompanied by easily being exhausted, rapid mood sways and palpitations appear. Most men report their erectile dysfunction as the most notable event during andropause. Apart from this, Dr. Tan's patients also complained of their being nervous, irritable and depressed.

Palpitations are due to the decrease of the testosterone level caused by over reaction of the autonomic system. It must be noted that it is natural for men who are suffering from andropause.

Formerly active men who used to be directed to their careers and power enhancement suddenly become close to family and their friends. However, there are some who preferred to find a new set up on their lifestyle which will turn them from the confusion and depression of andropause period.

The medical science has prepared remedies to relieve these symptoms. The problem is that most men do not submit to seeing a doctor even for health reasons. The reason is that it hits their masculine pride to be thought of as either vulnerable or dependent. This becomes a challenge to most wives.

One way to convince men to see the doctor is by accompanying him to a trained and understanding expert. By going together, the doctor can fully extract the needed information from the couple. However, there will also be times when the interview would be held independently to do away with the inhibitions.

As part of the clinical study, the following things are being checked as andropause basis: hair loss, shrinkage of testicles, decrease of libido and sex drive, erectile dysfunction, exhaustion, depression, decrease of muscle strength, oligospermia, and decrease in bone density.

Since the andropause stage could be very stressful among men, it is advisable that wives should become more understanding and supportive. Andropausal men should be encouraged to organize himself, to manage his alcohol and cigarette consumption, to relax, to eat healthy foods and to exercise.

Andropause is another profound journey which needs the positive involvement of the family. Not only men shall beat the odds, but everyone who loves him.

Unraveling the Truth about Andropause

For years, people have been hearing and learning about menopause and how to deal with it. Men and women are educated about this natural condition that affects women when they reach a certain age in order to properly cope with it and accept it as a natural condition.

However, another particular condition similar to menopause affects men and is a mystery on why this condition happens. This male menopause condition is called the andropause. Andropause is a condition that affects men that is very similar to women's menopause.

This condition is caused by low testosterone level in men and is considered as the male menopause condition that is affecting men when they reach a certain age. In the early 50s, andropause is defined as the natural cessation of sexual function in older men.

The symptoms of andropause relates very closely to menopause. It will include fatigue, depression, decreased sexual activity, and irritability. Surprisingly, this change has been always ignored and is considered as a normal phase in a man's life. It may be a normal thing, but it doesn't mean that men should suffer greatly from this condition.

Researchers suggest that andropause is caused by excess alcohol intake, stress, overweight, vasectomy, lack of exercise and ageing. Because of this, researchers have also begun to seek treatment methods to reduce the effects of andropause.

One solution to the problem is the Testosterone Replacement Therapy or TRT. This treatment showed promising results in effectively relieving symptoms of andropause. Adding to that, it also restores health, sex drive, and potency. It will also include a sense of renewed vitality and virility when it is given to the right patient, at the right time and at the right doses.

You have to realize the fact that the natural tendencies of men in the early years of his life are concerned primarily on their career, money and power. Often, men ignore and neglect family and friends to focus more on career. However, in the later years when andropause sets in, men becomes more maternal, as if the men changes role from being fatherly to becoming motherly. Surprisingly, men don't even sense the changes themselves and women notice it more. Women often tell doctors about this condition that their husbands are going through.

In response to the falling testosterone levels in the body, andropausal men will experience night sweats, and palpitations.

When men who experiences the mentioned symptoms and visits their doctor, the doctor will usually check for andropause by examining the following:

- Loss of hair in the armpits and axilla
- Low sex drive
- Erectile dysfunction or impotence
- Shrinkage of testicles
- Decreased muscle strength
- Depression
- Constant fatigue or tiredness
- Low sperm count
- Decreased bone density

Aside from the testosterone treatment, men should take the necessary steps in order to decrease the overall effects of andropause. The first step in treatment is to accept the condition. Once men accepted the condition it will be easier for them to treat it.

The next step is to exercise, and teach them to control themselves by quitting smoking and not abuse alcohol. Since, the body is changing while people age, men who are andropausal should also learn to relax and rest well.

These are the things that men should do when they reach the andropausal phase in life. This condition is inevitable and will affect men as they reach a certain age. Better to accept it and live life to the fullest rather than complain of not looking good anymore or being unable to have sex anymore.

The enlightenment of men's predicament on aging

Andropause is a stage in man's life when there is a noticeable declination in his hormones. This usually occurs at the late 40's or early 50's. The declination of hormonal production extends until the eighties. During this period, physical, emotional, psychological and behavioral manifestations due to declination of hormones become more visible.

Dr. Robert S. Tan, a renowned geriatrician conducted a study about male andropause which he compacted in his book "The Andropause Mystery: Unraveling Truths about the Male Menopause". The book deals with the physical changes and psychological challenges met by andropausal men. It serves as an eye opener on how to treat such a dilemma.

Andropause symptoms vary from one person to another. It is generally affected by the health condition. However, in the study of Dr. Robert Tan, some men between fifty to seventy years old reported the following symptoms: erectile dysfunction, tiredness, sudden mood sways, night sweats and occasional palpitations.

Aside from the physical changes, psychological changes that challenged their masculinity are augmented during the andropausal years. A man, no matter what age he is, tends to struggle to prove his strong sexuality, composed emotions, intellectual mind, supreme courage, good productivity, and strong personality, character and behavior.

But what happens when he's in the andropausal years?

The testosterone level of a young man at the age of 15-30 is 1000ng/dl. When he reaches the andropausal stage, an alarming drop of up to 800ng/dl causes the many predicaments in his life.

Dr R. Tan observed that the decrease of testosterone makes andropausal men likely to be more in touch with their feminine side. They become more involved in domestic issues which they use to ignore. They are more attentive to their roles at home such as cooking, housekeeping and bonding with their children. They devote much time now for the family and pleasure rather than their business roles. In a sense, the decrease of testosterone level makes them gentler and more domesticated.

On the mental side, judgment becomes less sharp than they used to be during a man's early age. He loses his accuracy and sharp mind. On some cases, there are reports of impaired memory which can lead to dementia.

The andropausal years can be directed to the question of courage. Men who are in this condition have the tendency to become more conservative and less of a risk taker. Fear can easily stun them. While some men fear death, most andropausal men fear to be too dependent.

The next attack hits the pride of being productive. As a common knowledge, men ought to be dynamic, to be noticed for his achievements and efforts. The source of man's happiness can be rooted on being the firm foundation of the family. When he reaches the andropausal period, he feels his inability to support his family as well as to manage complex business.

Personality is not a constant thing. Especially for men who are in their andropausal years, they are more susceptible to trimming down their being impulsive, hyperactive and ambitious. Through the passing of time, male menopause has begun to be accepted as part of aging.

But with the help of medical science, there are useful strategies formulated to cope up with the changes brought about by andropause. Careful supervision of a trained physician is though advisable.

Chapter 2 - Beat Male Menopause - Testosterone Replacement Therapy

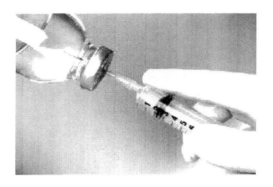

It is a fact that menopause is something that women will go though once they reach a certain age. During their late 40s, women experience this condition where their system will stop producing hormones. It is also a fact that menopause is often associated with women and few realize that it is also a condition where there is also a male counterpart of the menopause.

You may not know it but both male and female go through menopause. You may know about females going through menopause, but males going through the same condition are not really known and are still being debated as to the accuracy of the research.

The male menopause is caused by the decrease of the male's body capability to produce testosterone. Because of this, the signs and symptoms of male menopause can be compared closely to its female counterpart. Males who are going through this condition will experience getting depressed, irritable, and always getting tired or fatigued even with minimum movements such as walking from the front yard and back to the house.

Another symptom that you will see in a man who is going through male menopause is sexual disinterest. Because of this, it may affect his relationship with his spouse. It is known that many people who went through this stage in life have had problems with their marriage because of sexual disinterest.

This is why it is important for males and their wives to take all the necessary steps in treating this condition. Although male menopause occurs naturally once a man reaches a certain age, there are steps that couples can take to minimize the effects of male menopause.

Since one of the main causes of male menopause is the decrease of testosterone, the best way to treat or at least minimize the effects of the symptoms associated with male menopause is through testosterone replacement therapy. Through this therapy, you will be able to decrease the effects of symptoms, such as decreased interest in sex, depression and constant tiredness.

Because of this, you will be able to maximize your libido even if you are going through the condition of male menopause. This will significantly improve your sex life and also your social life with your partner. Through testosterone replacement therapy, not only will you be sexually active, but you can also improve your relationship with the people around you.

It is a fact that being irritable can cause a strain in your relationship with other people. By testosterone replacement therapy, you will be able to enjoy life once again, and decrease the risk of straining your relationship with other people.

Enjoy your manhood through testosterone replacement therapy. With this therapy, you will be able to cope up with male menopause and become a man again.

So, if you are ever experiencing what people call mid-life crisis, it is maybe because you are experiencing male menopause. You should always remember that menopause doesn't only occur on women, but it also occurs on the male population as well. You should also remember that this condition is natural and there is nothing you can do to stop it. The only thing you can do is minimize the symptoms through a therapy called testosterone replacement therapy or TRT. However, before you undergo TRT, you should always keep in mind that you should first consult your doctor. He or she will be able to recommend a clinic specializing in TRT with trained professionals to look after you.

Maximizing Manhood and Beating Male Menopause - Believe You Can

When a man reaches the age of 45, he started to worry of the next stage-death. Subsequently, his fear of being the next in line among his friends or relatives who had passed away drives him to do some silly things. And his tendency is to find more exciting things to venture on, just so he could hide the inactiveness and hormonal changes he's feeling inside.

That stage in man's life is called male menopause or andropause in medical terms.

Loss of vitality and fluctuation of virility level are the primary symptoms of andropause. This is due to the changes in production of the male sex hormones. In most cases, this predicament occurs at the age of 45 up to 55. But before the occurrence of andropause, there comes the mid-life crisis.

Dr. Malcolm Carruthers, the author of the book Maximizing Manhood: Beating male menopause explained the difference and occurrence of mid-life crisis and andropause.

These two distinct stages among males are often confused as one. In its real essence, these two are linked with each other since mid-life crisis happens between 35-45 years old right before the andropause period.

However, andropause comes early depending on how bad a man reacts to his mid-life crisis. Or, that it could be delayed if he had sustained a healthy and active lifestyle before this period.

Other signs of andropause include the abnormal drop of energy level, becoming more irritable, loss of sex drives and depression. Although some would consider these instances normal due to aging, you can still do something to overcome these effects. In medicine, andropause had grown to be a problem rather than a stage in life. For this reason, medical science has formulated solutions to this crisis.

Testosterone replacement therapy is formulated to relieve the symptoms of andropause among men. TRT comes in capsule, cream, implant or hormone patch forms. There are also claims for the efficiency of pills that contain male hormones and which can also relieve the symptoms of andropause. For those where neither of these works, pellet implant is also advisable. Testosterone pellets are implanted under the skin of the buttocks. The choice of which depends on how your body reacts to it. See which will work for you best.

The crisis in man's life called andropause is neither inherited nor natural for all men. Unlike that inevitable period among women called menopause, andropause can be beaten.

According to Carruther's study, there are external factors affecting the declination of testosterone level. Commonly, men living a healthy lifestyle decline in testosterone level by 1% yearly when he reaches the age of 40 to 70. This decrease of testosterone is more manifested among the unhealthy men.

Another factor which triggers the symptoms is stress. Both psychological and physical stresses which resorted to too much alcohol and cigarette consumption had aggravated the symptoms. In most cases, effects of malnutrition or nutritional deficiency are accounted to andropause. Symptoms such as anxiety, loss of memory and low sex drive could be due to aging or deficiency of chromium.

So examining it closely, not all men could suffer the effects of andropause. Such crisis is a big insult to a male body. And staying healthy, especially as you age, is a powerful weapon to overcome male menopause.

More Symptoms Associated With Male Menopause

Everyone knows that menopause is associated with women who reach a certain age. However, not many people are aware that menopause will also be experienced by the male population when they also reach a certain age. The male menopause condition or also known as andropause is very real and as a male, you have to be informed about it in order to cope with it. Male menopause occurs when you reach the age of about 50 to early 60's. The signs and symptoms of male menopause are quite similar to what women experience when they are going through the menopause.

However, unlike the female menopause where the production of hormones stops instantly, the male menopause will only decline in the production of male hormones called testosterone. This decline will result in the different signs and symptoms that you will experience when you go through male menopause. Male menopause will have symptoms similar to menopause that women experience, such as fatigue, infertility, hot flashes, and mood swings. However, there are more symptoms that men should be aware of when they experience male menopause.

You have to consider that you will also experience erectile dysfunction, loss of interest in sex, depression, and anxiety. There are also other symptoms linked to male menopause. Some men reported that they became more motherly. It is a fact that males are more focused on money, power, and career. When they experience male menopause, they somewhat reported that they became more focused on family, and friends, which is the primary concerns of women. Sometimes they say that they regretted their former attitude.

Males will also experience loss of hair in the armpits and axilla, decreased sex drive, shrinking of testicles, impotence, constant feeling of tiredness, decreased muscle strength, decreased muscle mass, decreased bone density, and low sperm count. All these symptoms points to male menopause. This is all due to the loss of androgens in the male's body. This is why there is testosterone replacement therapy as a treatment for men who are going through male menopause. It has been found that testosterone replacement can significantly improve your condition and decrease the signs and symptoms of male menopause.

There are also other treatments that are not as complicated as testosterone replacement therapy that you can do in order to improve your condition. However, it is recommended that you should mix these activities with testosterone replacement therapy. It is recommended that men should relax and rest well, exercise, eat the right kinds of food, and abstain from drinking and smoking.

Together with testosterone replacement therapy, you will see that it will significantly improve your condition. You will see that it will increase your sex drive or your libido, increase your muscle mass and strength, increase bone density, and it will also prevent depression.

Before you jump up and get yourself treated with testosterone replacement therapy, it is very important that you should consult your doctor first. The doctor will be able to determine if you have a low testosterone level by conducting a series of tests. The doctor will also be the one to recommend you to a qualified professional to do the testosterone replacement therapy.

Always remember that testosterone replacement therapy will not cure male menopause. It can only relieve the symptoms you experience associated with male menopause and can help you cope up with this condition. Just remember the signs and symptoms of male menopause and you can easily determine if you need to visit your doctor.

More Symptoms of Male Menopause

The condition and the symptoms of male menopause are comparable to the ones women experience and can sometimes be as worse. However male menopause does not affect all men, at least not with the same inclusion. Only some of the men between the age of forty and fifty can experience the condition and most of the symptoms of male menopause.

All the changes that occur in every man during the male menopausal period can affect every aspect of their lives. Male menopause is recognized as a physical condition and manifests in personal, psychological, social and spiritual dimensions.

Men also experience difficulties in hormonal fluctuations that affect their sexuality, mood, and personality like women. It is only one of the manifestations of the aging process of a man, where changes comes and make the person better out of it.

All men going through male menopausal can experience hormonal changes that greatly affect their lives. The levels of hormones will lower at their mid-life and may have changes which are usually associated with male menopausal. It is important to mark that every man has a unique personality and their individual levels of hormonal loss may vary widely. They have different outlook in life and strategies of living with satisfaction.

If the level of hormones lowers, it can be the cause to the decrease in sex drive and the general well being of their health. The occurrence of these things will also lead to the increase of depression and weight gain and absolutely will change the day to day living as compared to their lives before the onset of male menopause. During the menopausal period, some men can experience problems with regards to impotence. Wherein it is the constant inability to achieve and maintain an erection that is enough to have a satisfactory sexual performance. And because of impotency, men are having lowered sexual desires.

How can a man recognize that he is going through that certain stage in life, the menopausal period? There are some symptoms to be aware of. Some are physical, some are psychological, and some are sexual. The following are the symptoms that a male is going through a male menopausal period. Physical symptoms of male menopause include:

- Recovery from injuries and illness takes longer
- Less endurance for physical activity
- Gaining weight
- Difficulty reading small print
- Loss or thinning of hair
- Sleep disturbances
- Low libido
- Lack of energy

Psychological symptoms of male menopause include:

- Irritability
- Hesitancy or difficulty in making decisions
- Worry and fear for life
- Depression
- Having low self-esteem, self-confidence and joy
- Loss of purpose and direction in life
- Feeling alone, unattractive, and unloved
- Lack of memory and complexity in concentrating
- Mood swings

Sexual symptoms of male menopause include:

- Decreased sex drive
- Fear of sexual impotency

- More relationship problems and fights occurs with regards to sex, love, and intimacy
- Incapacity to erect during intimacy
- Increased of attraction to a much younger opposite sex

All the symptoms that a male can experience during the male menopausal period can be treated. Although men have been suffering from either physical, emotional or sexual symptoms of male menopause, you need to control it not through attempting self-diagnosis but by talking to a doctor, this will lead to being better informed and getting the proper treatment to alleviate the symptoms of the condition.

Overcome Male Menopause with Testosterone Treatment

There are facts today that supports that women are not the only ones who can suffer from changing hormones related to aging. It has been found that men too can suffer from the same symptoms that women experience during menopause. The so-called male menopause is still being debated whether they exist or not. However, evidence suggests that male menopause is very plausible and many males in society are suffering from this condition.

Also called andropause, the male menopause condition affects every male. This condition is natural and symptoms can be seen when men reach the age of late forties or early fifties. It has been found that when men age, the production of androgen declines. Because of the decrease of androgen, males suffer from male menopause with some symptoms that are very similar to menopause that occurs on women. Men that are undergoing androgen decline or andropause experience constant fatigue and weakness, depression, and also sexual problems.

However, unlike in women where hormone production stops completely, the male hormone or the testosterone declines in a much slower process. This means that men who are healthy can still be able to produce sperm even if he already reached the age of eighty or even longer. The male menopause will have devastating effect to men and their spouses. This is because with decreased sexual activity and constant irritability, it will likely result in an unhealthy relationship within the marriage. Because of this, many couples undergo marriage counseling at this age and sometimes, men who goes through this condition goes into depression.

However, there are available treatments today that can decrease the signs and symptoms of male menopause. In fact, this kind of treatment will improve sexual health and also social well-being of males who are going through the male menopause stage. This treatment is called the testosterone replacement therapy or TRT. This revolutionary treatment will help males who are experiencing the male menopause condition accept it better. The treatment will be able to relieve some of the symptoms associated with the male menopause condition, such as depression, loss of interest in sex, and constant tiredness or fatigue.

The testosterone replacement therapy is available in oral, IV, and patch forms. This particular treatment should always be done with a professional in order to give the patient the proper dose of testosterone to avoid any unwanted side effects and also to increase the benefits that males can get with the therapy. Through this therapy, males and their spouses will be able to live a happier and healthier life. If your spouse is suffering from male menopause, it is likely that he won't notice the signs and symptoms. Try to tell them about this condition and recommend the testosterone replacement therapy as an answer to his problems.

With this therapy, it will be able to decrease the symptoms associated with male menopause. It will decrease the feeling of depression, and constant tiredness or fatigue, and it will significantly increase the sex drive of males. However, before undergoing such treatment, you and your spouse should first consult your doctor first. The doctor will run a series of tests in order to determine if testosterone replacement therapy is the right choice. The doctor will also be able to recommend testosterone replacement therapy specialists who will be able to assist you and your spouse during the therapy sessions.

Chapter 3 - A Guide in Surviving Male Menopause for Men and Women

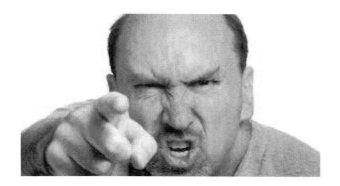

The male menopause or andropause is a condition that all men will go through once they reach a certain age. It is something that everybody should know how to deal with, especially men and their spouse.

This condition is very similar to female's menopause condition where there are also related symptoms. The cause of andropause or male menopause is the decline of hormones as they age.

If you think men are spared from menopause, you should think again. The andropause condition or the male menopause condition will eventually affect all men once they reach a certain age. This particular condition is associated with the decline of male hormone levels that occurs at certain age, usually when men reach late 40's or early 50's.

The main symptoms of andropause are erectile dysfunction or failure to achieve erection, mood changes, night sweats, constant fatigue or tiredness, and also irritability and depression. Some even said that when men are suffering from andropause, they become more motherly than fatherly. They tend to be focused more on family and friends rather than the natural focus of men on money, career, and power in the early life before the andropausal stage.

Surprisingly, the change isn't always noticed by men who are going through the andropausal stage. The men's spouses do notice it and have constantly said that their husbands are going through the menopause.

There will also be physical changes associated with andropause, such as loss of hair in the armpits and axilla, shirking of the testicles, lessening of muscle mass, and also decreased muscle strength.

This change is due to the loss of androgens in a man's body. Androgen's is known to be the basic ingredient that makes up masculinity and because of the loss of this ingredient, physical change occurs.

Andropause may cause depression in men and because of their irritability; it may also cause depression in their spouses. This is why it is important for women to know how to deal with andropause and teach their husbands to know how to deal with it too. Here are some ways women can teach their husbands to cope up with the inevitable changes that andropause can cause:

- The first thing a woman should teach her husband is to teach them how to love and reward themselves as well as love and reward others.

- Men are usually abusive when it comes to alcohol and smoking. Teach men not to abuse alcohol and also quit smoking at the same time. Tell them that it will lessen the signs and symptoms of andropause or male menopause and also, will be healthier for them.

- Lack of exercise is a known cause of early aging. This is why it is important to encourage men to exercise. This will prolong their youth and also slow down the physical changes that naturally occurs when people age.

- Eating right is also one of the best ways to combat andropause. Teach men to eat qualitatively and not quantitatively. Tell them that it is more important to eat the right kind of food instead of eating more of the wrong kinds of food.

- Andropause is inevitable and will eventually happen as men reach a certain age. Teach your husband to deal with it. Teach them to accept it in order to live life to the fullest. Tell them to seek out some hobby in order for them to take their mind off the condition.

These are some of the ways you can effectively help your husband when they are suffering from andropause. Always remember that this condition is unavoidable and it is relatively the same as menopause. The best thing you can do is accept it and enjoy it.

Surviving Male Menopause

Jed Diamond is a licensed psychotherapist practicing his profession for almost 40 years. He is also the director of the health program MenAlive which aims in helping men to live well and live long. He has already authored seven books which include the best seller "Male Menopause" which is translated into fourteen languages and "Surviving Male Menopause" containing other important factors of a man's life discussed in details.

For Jed Diamond, it is very important to understand the andropause phenomenon which occurs in men. As this brought physiological and psychological changes, affected people might get really upset and their family members may also suffer the consequences. This is true especially for married people. In general, wives carry the burden of their changed husband. They also get confused and despaired about their husband's personality especially when talking about moods and attitudes.

"Surviving Male Menopause" educates women regarding the most complicated stage of the men's life. The book contains eight chapters which are easy to understand. It is a complete book which discusses about male menopause on a more personal outlook. Women also speak their side as they gain a deeper understanding of what the phenomenon really is. It is true that some women who lack understanding can be blown off against what their husbands has been showing to them jeopardizing their marital relationship.

Hear stories from men revealing the truth as they experienced a complicated biological change in their lives. Maybe your mind is bombarded by a lot of questions regarding male menopause but afraid to know it. Well, in this book you will find the answers. It is a fact that before facing their later years, men once become adolescents and more mature during their middle age. The stages of manhood are thoroughly discussed providing guidelines on how to survive each stage.

Men could hardly accept it that andropause is striking them. They face their greatest fear thus denying that apparent symptoms of andropause in them are not happening. How can anyone accept the fact that they are losing their energy, sex drive and physical agility? Moreover, they would also deny that IMS (Irritable Male Syndrome) is attacking them. It is the condition wherein sudden mood swings occurs from once being lovable, contented, and peaceful to becoming mean, discontented, and agitated. In this book, men are taught how to overcome their fear and denial stage.

Male menopause has different factors to deal with. Men can never successfully pass this stage without proper knowledge of how to get through it. As some mostly believe that it is the end of men's sexual power. But if they would follow the right direction then it is worth in the end conquering defeating consequences. Remember, that looking ahead with a good disposition can help. Male menopause is only a passage to a more passionate, purposeful, and productive time in men's life.

Experiencing and passing the male menopausal stage can probably bring in useful benefits. "Surviving Male Menopause" truly serves a guide for both men and women to achieve peace and harmony in their relationship despite its effects. Jed Diamond ensures that men's menopause should not threaten the couple's future to live happily like before. Changes are normal, but most people differ in their view of acceptance. Take note, men and women who are more educated will have a higher percentage of survival.

Chapter 4 - Male Menopaws: The Silent Howl

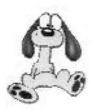

When males reach the age of late 40's or early 50's, they will somewhat experience a condition called the mid-life crisis. They tend to get depressed, tend to get conscious with their appearance and they tend to have little interest in sex.

This condition is also called the male menopause where the testosterone level found in males declines and causes them to get depressed, irritable, experience constant tiredness or fatigue and also cause them to have decreased interest in sex. In some cases, males become impotent when they reach this age.

This is why there are self-help books such as the Male Menpaws: The Silent Howl written by Marty Sacks and Jack Davis to help males all over the world overcome the mid-life crisis. This book is designed to inform and teach males to cope up with the difficulties that a middle-aged man experiences.

This book also has illustrations of gentleman dogs that offer humorous solutions for the difficulties of middle-aged males experience in today's society. If you are a female, this book is a great gift for your husband who is reaching or who has reached that certain age where he often gets depressed. This book will be able to inform him gently about the facts of life and that life is what you make of it.

This book informs men gently about the harshness of change and it also contains how to cope up with it. This book will tell them to stop pouting and move on with their lives in a humorous way to make it easier for males to accept it.

It is a fact that changes in life as you age can be harsh. It can affect both men and women and this change in physical and emotional state is inevitable and should be accepted in order to better cope up with it.

The Male Menopaws: The Silent Howl offers comprehensive information about the truth about aging and ways to help you overcome the mid-life crisis stage in life. This is where males will learn how to make the most of it and will also help them learn more about themselves.

It is a fact that not many males will be willing to accept the fact that they are growing older every day. This book will help them accept that fact and accept it with pride.

So, if you ever have a friend who is suffering from mid-life crisis or if you have a spouse who is also suffering from mid-life crisis, try and purchase this book for them. You have to consider the fact that they won't be buying this book anytime soon. So, it would definitely be a good idea if you give this book to them as a gift.

They will surely enjoy reading it and at the same time, make them realize that being middle-age is not that bad at all. You will see that after they have read this book, they will be more mature and they will also accept what they have naturally become in life.

This book is a must-read for every male who is going through the dreaded mid-life crisis where they often get depressed and very conscious on how they appear. With this book, they will be more confident about themselves and accept the aging process better.

Menopause--The Silent Howl for Males

An aged man walks along the road when a frog shows up in all of a sudden, the frog uttered to him, "If you will kiss me I will transform into a beautiful maiden." The man, after hearing the words of the frog, picks it up at once and places it inside of his purse. The frog in its great confusion asked the man, "Why didn't you kiss me?" But the man answers, "I would prefer to have a frog talking inside of my purse."

This story can be likened to a satire wherein it depicts an aged man with a sexual insecurity. According to some researches, a man reaching the age of 50 and 60 are already not capable to perform for quite several reasons. And this situation is often associated to male menopause.

Nowadays, approximately 18 million of the male American population is affected with this dilemma on waning sexual potency, affected by the lowering of the testosterone level.

Moreover, this dilemma which is often termed as the midlife crisis for aging men does not solely affect their sexual potency; this also affects their mood, as well as their endurance, quite akin to the feelings of women when they are also reaching their menopausal period.

According to specialists, male menopausal may show various symptoms like frequent fatigue, grouchiness, the lowering of sex drive, decrease in life's enjoyment, waning strength of erections, falling fast asleep after eating dinner, the ability in sports is gradually declining, lowering of strength and stamina, and decrease in energy.

If a man above the age of 50 is experiencing three of the mentioned symptoms, there is a chance that it might already be a low testosterone syndrome.

There are statistical studies that also reveal the effects that can be related to the lowering of testosterone level, these are:

- Reduce of libido level; this includes the eagerness for sex and the sexual thoughts
- Reduce in muscle mass
- Reduce of memory level
- Increase of heart ailments

It is usual that on the part of the women, they often perceive that men will not go through to anything like what they will go through as they reach their midlife.

However, with all these presented facts about male menopausal, it shows that women and men will be going through to a closely alike experience in the later years of their lives.

People frequently focus on the differences between the menopause of male and female that they tend to neglect the numbers of its similarities, like for instance the impulsive mood swings, anxiety and bad temper, the aching of neck and back, the lapses and loses of memory, the lowering of concentration, lowering of self-esteem, the feeling of gaining weight, and sickness or injury takes longer time to cure.

Although men go through some reproductive modification, they do not lose their capacity for reproduction, unlike women. However, because men are considered to have a sturdy performance in terms of sex, many of these men would prefer to keep the frog talking inside of his purse and dismiss the fact that it can transform into a beautiful maiden, than let the situation caused by male menopause insult his sexuality.

Note this, the fatigue brought by male menopausal dilemma is taken by these men quietly, yet, inside of them there is an out bursting howl.

Chapter 5 - Mr. Hyde and Dr. Jekyll Syndrome vs. Male Menopause

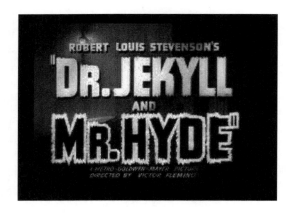

Adams descendant, the male species is unpopularly known to be afflicted with a critical illness – Dr. Jekyll and Mr. Hyde Syndrome or the Male Menopause.

Dr. Jekyll and Mr. Hyde Syndrome

In 1886, Robert Stevenson wrote a book about Dr. Jekyll and Mr. Hyde wherein he discussed the quest of Dr. Jekyll to divide the two characters of human so that he can separately define good from evil. No individual during his time supported Dr. Jekyll's experiment hence he performed the test upon himself, which gave birth to Mr. Hyde, the evil side of Dr. Jekyll.

Mr. Hyde started his revenge to all the people who disheartened Dr. Jekyll. The madness, misery and vengeance were all over. Mr. Hyde is uncontrollable. His wickedness is unstoppable. Dr. Jekyll had so many struggles controlling his evil part, Mr. Hyde.

Male Menopause

Male menopause or sometimes referred to as andropause is a condition where a man goes through an unavoidable change in social, interpersonal, psycho-logical and even the spiritual aspect.

Similarity of Dr. Jekyll and Mr. Hyde Syndrome with Male Menopause

Both Dr. Jekyll and Mr. Hyde Syndrome and Male Menopause are considered transitional stages of men.

Dr. Jekyll had longings to separate the good identity from the evil one. This may be explained to man's desire to be completely good or entirely bad which most of the time are dictated by events in human's life. Men are faced in an intersection where they have to decide the path they need to take – the good or the bad one.

Male menopause, on the other hand, is a shift from first adulthood to second adulthood. It is commonly described as the maturation of men wherein they focused more on the inner self, compared to the previous stage of his life where he is much focused with the outer being.

Differences between Male Menopause and Dr. Jekyll and Mr. Hyde Syndrome

Dr. Jekyll and Mr. Hyde syndrome differs with male menopause in terms of the following:

? Dr. Jekyll and Mr. Hyde syndrome can happen to men anytime. It knows no age. On the other hand, male menopause usually takes place when a man is about to reach second adulthood, it can emerge as early as thirty-five years old or as late as sixty-five.

? Male menopause is highly associated as a hormonal or chemical change, which may have a positive or negative effect towards the whole being of a man. While Dr. Jekyll and Mr. Hyde syndrome is more of a psychological change. Additionally, the triggering factor is primarily environmentally related such as overexposure to vices, influences of friends or misfortunes in life.

Most of the time, the syndrome portrays negative effect unless the evil part has been defeated. The abovementioned conditions can make or break a man. If Mr. Hyde rules, a man's life then peace and love will not have a room in his heart. Not only will a man suffer but also his family will significantly be affected. If Dr. Jekyll's personality will govern then negative emotions may not be felt or even expressed which then can affect both the individual and his significant others. There should be a Dr. Jekyll and Mr. Hyde in the life of a man, so that there will be balance.

Male menopause can break a man if he perceive and acts negatively on the said condition. The condition can help him achieve the man he ought to be if the male species will have a positive attitude towards andropause.

Surviving and understanding the Jekyll and Hyde male menopause syndrome

Some if not all men fear this certain stage in man's life called male menopause. For many, this crisis is the start of half dying and half living nature. But what about male menopause is really scary? When a man reaches the age of 40, he starts to become irritable, easily stressed and starts to lose his passion and purpose in life. This turning point of the way to andropause haunted men in one way or another - Male menopause syndrome.

There are three causes linked to male menopause syndrome. First is the fluctuation of male hormones. This is a normal occurrence as we age. But also, this can be manifested due to lack of nutrients and exercise. The next factor is the change in the brain's biochemistry. The decrease in the supply of neurotransmitters increases hostility, anger and impatience. The third and the resolvable cause is the increase of stress level. It could be due to too much consumption of alcohol or due to psychological stresses. How you handle circumstances can be a big factor in this area. It could be avoided if only you would try. These factors became part of the mid-life struggles which challenge men to overcome.

Many wives had their stories to tell about their partners with altering characters, husbands who turn from being Jekyll to Hyde, from being compassionate to mean. The male menopause syndrome patterned to the book of Robert Louis Stevenson entitled "Dr. Jekyll and Mr. Hyde" had so much in common.

The story is about Dr. Jekyll who had this pursuit of separating the good and the bad nature of man. In his quest, he encountered rejections from colleagues and superiors. For that he had to work alone for his project. Then, Dr. Jekyll had to do the experiment with himself. That separated his evil nature who turned out to be Mr. Hyde. In contrary to the good persona of Dr. Jekyll, Mr. Hyde had been murdering the board of governors who turned down the cause of Dr Jekyll. All through the story, Dr Jekyll had been pursuing in vain to control his evil half.

The same pursuit happens to men who are suffering from the male menopause syndrome. From being the responsible and loving Jekyll, they had the tendency to turn to being the irritable Hyde. Men at this age seemed to change overnight. But these tendencies are often triggered by loss of a friend or relative. The death of a close person seemed to trigger thoughts of them being the next in line. And the realization of their being mortal is so striking that he has convoluted thoughts. The confusion that he feels is often accounted to his responsibilities and to the people surrounding him. Then he describes this feeling as being trapped and subsequently loses his sense of being.

At this crisis, men need to be understood. It is a crucial period when a man would want to be free and to destroy the order of the old ways. It is the period when they need to feel needed, and that they are important. There could be a lot of remedies in store trying to relieve the symptoms of male menopause. They can cause side effects, however. The best cure is to give them enough support and guidance to overcome this crisis.

Understanding the Jekyll Hyde Male Menopause Syndrome

Andropause is a condition brought about by low levels of testosterone throughout the man's body. It normally occurs in men aged 40 years old and above where they experience symptoms similar to women's menopause. However, changes in men are gradual, characterized by fatigue, changes in moods and attitudes, and loss of physical agility, energy, and sex drive. Studies show that men may even acquire the Jekyll Hyde Syndrome or Irritable Male Syndrome (IMS) which can later on affect the people around him.

A lot of people are familiar with the book written by Robert Louis Stevenson entitled Dr. Jekyll and Mr. Hyde. It speaks about human psyche dealing with the mind of a male in particular. Dr. Henry Jekyll has a life-long pursuit of separating man's two natures to obtain the essence between evil and good.

Dr. Jekyll superiors and friends refused to help him. However, he succeeded in doing his experiments using his formula, but the results were shocking. Dr. Jekyll's evil nature, Edward Hyde, surfaces with a separate identity. Hyde starts to murder those people who refuse to support Dr. Jekyll's cause. From then on, Dr. Jekyll keeps on fighting to control his evil half.

It is really shocking that this transformation could occur with men undergoing andropause. Their attitudes can suddenly change from being once a loving and sensitive person to becoming mean and uncaring. Some wife does complain to their husbands that they completely changed from being Dr. Jekyll to Mr. Hyde.

There are pointers to understand in the manifestation of this syndrome. Mostly, men who experience IMS can really change apparently overnight. He could appear so peaceful, loving, and contented but suddenly he freaks out as agitated, mean, and discontented. Other factor which triggers the condition involves a crisis of a relative or close friend. It could also be a difficulty in achieving his real identity since he has different roles such as being a father, a son, a husband, or a friend. This leads to confusion and fear thinking that he has to destroy his old version to move into something new.

IMS has affected a lot of men. It was mentioned earlier that plummeting testosterone levels can cause a man to become withdrawn and irritable which is considered an internal cause. However, external causes also trigger IMS in men. It can include physical injury or illness, or a relationship or job loss. So he thinks that his problems are caused by another person thus complaining more about it. Then he justifies it with anger to release the blame viewing the world via distorted lenses.

But not all men acquired IMS. There are four factors that should come together to develop IMS. It is determined by changes in hormones, brain chemistry, loss of identity, and stress levels. You just can't easily rate men who are irritable and angry with IMS. They should take the tests to be sure that they have IMS since being irritable and angry are normal.

Men can seek counseling to treat IMS so that they could prevent themselves from becoming Mr. Hyde of course. Men having low levels of testosterone can have testosterone restoration. Right diet and exercise is also significant. Exercising can increase testosterone levels. But keep in mind that low-carb diets are not helpful. Low carbohydrates can lower serotonin levels making men irritable. Remember, understanding IMS and seeking proper help is worth all the effort.

Chapter 6 - Male Menopause Phase

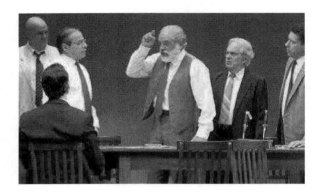

Hormonal change – two words which can bring significant change to an individuals' life. Once hormonal change is brought into discussion, most people would correlate it to women. These days however, women are not the only ones who experience hormonal change, men as well.

Menopause is the normal and natural stage in a woman's life when her menstruation and ovulation ceases that signifies end to her reproductive years. On the other hand, andropause is a term for male menopause. Since a man does not undergo menstruation and ovulation, the reason behind for male experiencing menopause is to prepare them for second adulthood. Andropause signifies the end for men's first adulthood.

Women who enter their forties may begin to experience menopause. Other women starts menopause at age fifty, some even begin at sixty. Men, on the other hand, may start to undergo andropause as early as thirty-five or it can be as late as sixty-five. While female menopause is a start for women to feel unconstructive sentiments and other pessimistic emotions, most experts believe that andropause brings positive change.

A man will go through a crucial change once he enters the andropause stage. There is inevitable change in psychological, social, interpersonal and even the spiritual aspect. Andropause denotes "the end of the beginning." According to research, there are a lot of benefits a man can obtain once andropause is experienced.

Maturity is the essential benefit of man in going through male menopause. Men on their first adulthood usually focus on doing. However this time as they enter the second adulthood, they are more focused with "the being," or "the self." Career-wise, they are more inclined to accomplish their job because of "love of work" instead of going to work because it is necessary. On social relationship, men tend to look at other men as acquaintances. During first adulthood, men interact with other men as contenders.

A man's personal relationship also matures. He is more focused with developing happiness and intimacy with his partner. Andropause may indicate a stop in brain-draining "battle of the sexes" which may be an indication that he can give way and make his partner win on some discussion. Ego and pride are left behind. It is transformed to in-depth understanding and patience. Men also gains maturity in a sexual relationship. Second adulthood focuses more on being sexually fulfilled compared to concentrating on different sexual performances which usually takes place during first adulthood.

Menopause is a period in life where an individual may start to feel incomplete. Others may accordingly react to what their body dictates. Good or bad – whatever menopause may create in one's life, you are still the one who owns your mind, body and heart. If andropause brings you more benefit, then you are of the lucky few. Otherwise, if it creates struggles in your life then it is time to acknowledge the need for help. Primarily, you need to recognize that you are undergoing change and then let your significant other know about it. Point out the necessary things they must do to help you cross the line. If things seem unbearable after exhausting all possible help within your fence, then it is time to seek help from an expert. A successful walk in the journey of male menopause boils down to one important thing, having good attitude.

Male Menopause Enlarged

There are currently numerous debates in the medical community on whether menopause really exists in men. Menopause in women is defined as the time when the menstrual periods cease. Based on this, men cannot have menopause. But, as the doctors have argued, they can undergo andropause — the male equivalent of menopause in women. Male who have andropause manifest the same symptoms as those women with menopause.

Male menopause is used to refer to the condition in which men experience a decrease in their hormone levels. But unlike the case of women whose hormone levels drop dramatically, male menopause takes place with a gradual fall in hormone testosterone. Medical reports show that many men in their 70's have almost the same testosterone levels as those in their 20's.

Men with menopause manifest symptoms that include irritability, sweating, memory problems, concentration difficulties, and hot flushing. Other common complaints of men with menopause consist of low sex drive, hair loss, fatigue, generalized pains, and body shape changes as they tend to become more rounded and less brawny.

Analyzing the symptoms, it becomes clear why male menopause is compared with that of women. Women may manifest some or all of the symptoms listed.

It is important to note, however, that the symptoms listed may be caused by other physical illnesses other than menopause. Thyroid gland dysfunction, depression, or anemia may be the underlying roots.

Some doctors, however, claim that male menopause is caused not by the hormonal changes but by psychological reasons. The realization that they are ageing is underlined by the signs of physical changes such as the occurrence of wrinkles, fat and waning hairline.

Men in their middle age usually weaken their self-esteem as they begin to question themselves as to whether they still have a role in their homes and the society. An example is when their children mature and leave home; they start to feel empty and futile in the family.

Other possible psychological triggers of menopause in men include financial problems, job dissatisfaction, and marital conflicts.

It is important to note, however, that the symptoms listed may be caused by other physical illnesses other than menopause. Again, thyroid gland dysfunction, depression, or anemia may be the underlying causes.

The diagnosis of male menopause is done by running a physical exam; the doctor will inquire about the symptoms the male is experiencing. He may conduct necessary diagnostic tests to discard other medical problems which may be affecting the condition. Series of blood tests will then be carried out to analyze the patient's hormone levels, as well as the blood testosterone status.

Testosterone replacement therapy is applied if the testosterone levels are found to be low. This process also helps to minimize the symptoms such as fatigue, depression, and low libido, or poor sex drive.

Hormone replacement therapy has as well been tied to the development in the brain functions, bone density and night sweats.

Testosterone replacement comes in oral medication, implants, or injections. The oral drugs are given to those who cannot bear implants or injections. On the other hand, implants are placed in the lower hip or abdomen.

This method provides cure that keeps going for up to six months. The testosterone injections are typically given about once every two weeks.

If you are considering testosterone replacement therapy, it is important that you talk to a doctor to learn more about it. Your physician may also advise some changes in your lifestyle, such as an exercise program, proper diet, and medications to help alleviate the symptoms caused by male menopause.

Chapter 7 - Male Menopause and Depression

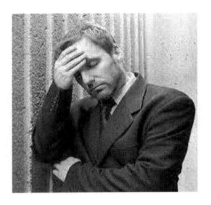

You may not know it but men also experiences a certain condition that many thought only women experiences. This condition can get someone depressed and lose interest in sex. This condition is called male menopause.

For years, many people have always linked menopause to women. However, studies have found that males also experience this condition. Sometimes, people describe this condition as mid-life crisis. Male menopause has been found to have similar symptoms that women experience.

Male menopause occurs when a man reaches a certain age. When you reach the late 50's to early 60's, you will see that you will experience male menopause. One of the known symptoms of male menopause is depression. Males who experience this condition will be constantly sad, anxious and depressed. Because of this, it may be mistaken for depression.

However, because of the decline in testosterone levels in men who experience male menopause, depression will occur. You have to consider that male menopause will also cause anxiety and loss of interest in sex.

This is why you should think about getting male menopause treatment in order to alleviate the symptoms. One such treatment is called hormone replacement therapy for men. Usually, this treatment is done for men who have low testosterone level. However, because of male menopause and the decline of the body's production of testosterone, the testosterone replacement therapy is now done on men who are going through male menopause.

By going through this process when you are going through male menopause, it will significantly decrease the effects of male menopause. You have to consider the fact that testosterone replacement therapy will not cure male menopause. It will just help in alleviating the signs and symptoms associated with low testosterone level and male menopause.

Depression is one of the conditions of male menopause. By going through the testosterone replacement therapy, you will see that it will help you get rid of depression. It will also help you with your erectile dysfunction condition and will significantly improve your sex life. With testosterone replacement therapy, you will have your sex life back again.

However, before jumping in and get yourself treated with testosterone replacement therapy, you first have to consult with your doctor. The doctor will determine if you are indeed going through male menopause. By conducting a series of tests, the doctor will determine if your testosterone level has declined. If it has, the doctor will then recommend treatments, such as testosterone replacement therapy.

The doctor will be able to recommend a professional who is able to administer and supervise the treatment. You have to consider the fact that it is necessary for you to have the right dosage of testosterone in order to have maximum effect while getting rid of the side effects.

There are different ways that testosterone replacement therapy is done. There is the injection method, the oral capsules method, the patches method, and also the implant method. Professionals in testosterone replacement therapy will let you choose which method is right for you and which method you are most comfortable with.

Always remember that testosterone replacement therapy should only be done with the supervision of a qualified professional in the field of the testosterone replacement therapy. This is important in order to give you the best effect possible while minimizing or eliminating unwanted side effects.

So, get your life back on track, get rid of depression, and cope with male menopause through testosterone replacement therapy.

Male Menopause Symptoms and Its Strategies in Surviving Depression

It is not surprising that men are not spared from biological occurrences. Like women, men have also their menopausal stage. The male menopause known as andropause is a condition wherein the hormones of males naturally decline. Moreover, changes in their lives such as reordering life, career change, or divorce also happens. These events bring physiological and psychological changes which can later on become depression.

Andropause usually occurs in men at the age fifty and above. But some people are asking questions whether andropause is real or only a myth. Well, it is a fact that hormonal decline is not prevented as one person ages. However, the hormone declines in men are more gradual compared to women's menopause. That is why andropause is medically termed as A.D.A.M or Androgen Decline in Aging Males.

Like women's menopause, andropause in men are also characterized by different symptoms. These symptoms are apparent which are being manifested by erectile dysfunction or the failure of achieving an erection, mood changes, general tiredness, palpitations, and night sweats. Palpitations and night sweats happen because the autonomic system of men is overactive responding to their testosterone falling levels. But erectile dysfunction is considered the most important symptom of andropause.

Feelings to be closer to their family as well as friends are also developed during the andropause stage. Men in their early stage of life often focus on money, career, and power but when andropause strikes them, the transitions are clearly seen. These men became more concerned with their family and friends as if they regret their past attitudes.

Another symptom that is commonly reported is memory loss associated with the aging process. Nevertheless it is only minor and will not affect daily functioning compared to Alzheimer's disease.

As been said, andropause brings changes in men both physically and psychologically. Therefore, men should handle issues and changes carefully because these can cause stress. If stress is not successfully managed then depression might take place. But worry no more since there are six strategies so that men can successfully passed the andropause stage.

1. Learning to reward and love themselves and others. Remember that it is much better to give than to receive. It is very important to leave legacies.

2. Controlling and organizing their self. Keep in mind that discipline is vital as they face their later life. It is much better not to abuse themselves with alcohol and cigarettes. Time management is also good for preparing wills, advancing directives, and designating management.

3. Exercising. Muscle and cardiovascular conditioning surely helps in delaying aging processes.

4. Having good relaxation and rest periods. This is good for coping up with physiological changes.

5. Obtaining the right diet. Take note that it is necessary to eat foods suited to their age.

6. Enjoying the andropause and aging stage. Accept that there are inevitable things beyond human control. Learn to be satisfied and just make the most out of what life has to offer. Andropause is part of life's journey so be positive about it and concentrate on acquired blessings rather than being depressed.

Asking for the advice of a doctor can also help. Counseling may treat some physical and psychological changes. Fortunately, treatment for mood changes and erectile dysfunction or impotence is easily accessible today.

Men should take these helpful steps to avoid depression and see the brighter side of life despite facing andropause.

What You Can Do With Male Menopause and Depression

Men are considered tough. At a young age they were taught how to wear masks. Emotions, especially feelings, which denotes weakness does not have any room in a man's life. Men in effect tend to deny what they truly feel. Studies show that men are more susceptible to depression since negative emotions are suppressed.

Depression is an emotional disorder. An individual who is said to be depressed begins to experience prolonged sadness, time and again anxiety, inability to concentrate, unexplainable anger and low self-esteem.

The occurrence of depression varies. Some people experience it as a form of reaction to uneventful situations in their lives. Others feel depressed as a response to excessive smoking, drinking alcoholic beverages and taking drugs. Depression can also be inevitable when an individual undergoes chemical and hormonal changes in the body.

Male menopause or known as andropause to some, is a condition in which a man undergo changes – it may be physical, emotional, or to some extent spiritual. If a male individual reacts negatively towards andropause, then he is prone to experience depression.

"Boys don't cry," is a cliché. It is high time that men do what is necessary to fight depression caused by male menopause phenomenon.

Acknowledgement is a key to acceptance. Male individuals should acknowledge that they too like their female counterpart also experience menopause.

Education then leads to better understanding. After accepting the fact that you have male menopause then it is best to educate yourself with the said condition. Learn what the signs and symptoms are, then the diagnosis and treatments. It is also best if you undertake research for facts and issues concerning andropause. The Internet is a good venue to learn more about male menopause and depression. There are also online organizations which you can turn to that can help you with your dilemma.

Better understanding is a bridge for you to project a positive attitude. Negative emotions block your sensibility for you to have better comprehension of what is happening in your body. Depression usually roots to suppress negative emotions. It is not asked from you to portray a happy face yet you are miserable deep inside. What is being asked from you is that you have to learn how to deal with the situation. Make no room for self-pity for it will only worsen the situation.

Do something about it. After you have taken the necessary steps then move forward to getting help. Primarily, get help from your significant others. This is the time when their unconditional support and love is needed. Explain to them what you are going through. Let them know what specific help you need, if there are.

You can seek assistance from a physician who has expertise in andropause and depression. He can point out the changes that might happen to you and further prescribe you on what you should do.

Support groups may also be helpful. If there are support groups in your community, then it is best to join them so that you will feel that you are not alone in your battle.

No man should allow depression to rule his life. Male menopause is never a reason for you to wallow in depression. After all, look at the brighter side of things, andropause welcomes you to a new phase in your life – a phase where you can put down your mask and reveal your true self.

Chapter 8 - Testosterone Talk: Symptoms of Male Menopause

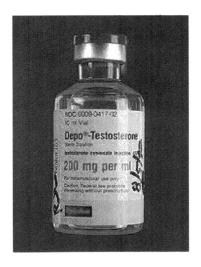

Shrugged shoulders – this is men's common reaction whenever menopause is discussed by their significant other. Perhaps the reaction can be taken into account with the fact that it is hard to understand something that you do not personally experience.

What if men experience menopause? Will they begin to understand a woman's menopausal plight?

It may be a resounding yes or no. Medical studies show that women are not the only ones who experience menopause, men does too. The term is referred to as male menopause commonly known as andropause. Viropause is another term for male menopause. This is described to be the cause of low testosterone levels. Others view it as an end to first adulthood and an indication to begin second adulthood. Some individuals on the other hand view andropause in a sexual manner, wherein it signifies deterioration of sexual desires and performance.

Men may find this fact alarming. Perhaps then, they will start to realize and later on comprehend how it is like to have drastic hormonal change. Menopause for women has distinct and defined symptoms such as stop of menstrual cycle, hot flashes which is evident on the face, chest and neck, too much perspiration, dryness in the vagina, throbbing heartbeat, body aches, itching skin, the growth of hair increases specifically on face but growth of hair decreases on armpit and pubic hair.

On the other hand, dropping of testosterone produced is the most well-defined symptom of male menopause. This can be screened and identified after consulting a physician since decrease in testosterone may also be associated with other illnesses such as diabetes. Once testosterone level has gone down, the following symptoms may be transparent:

- Physical exhaustion from simple tasks. The usual alertness and drive to easily accomplish tasks decreases. Being usually tired however does not contribute for a man to gain better sleep. At this stage, he may suffer from insomnia.
- Furthermore, increase in weight and body fat is evident yet unexplainable.
- Mental fatigue. The ability to concentrate lessens. He may need time to digest things being discussed

over a conversation, on a written material or even audio-related matters.
- Emotional exhaustion. At this time, a man's temper varies. He may feel happy now and suddenly sadness might strike him. Sadness aside, he may depict an angry attitude most of the time. Moreover, a man experiencing male menopause can easily be observed as always nervous.
- Decrease in sexual desire. This may be due to failure to get or sustain an erection.

Andropause is not an alarming situation if men have apt knowledge on facts about male menopause. It will also be helpful if he gains knowledge on its symptoms so he can gauge whether or not he is suffering from andropause. To further verify the condition, a visit to a physician is highly recommended.

The situation will be less distressing for men if their significant others will well support him. If women needs heightened support, love and understanding during the menopausal stage, men in the same way needs it.

Now that there is a male version of menopause, maybe then the successor of Adam will be able to understand what is going with a woman's body when she begins to experience menopause. Perhaps now there will be no more shrugging of shoulders. Instead there will be a shoulder to lean on hard times such as undergoing andropause.

Male Menopause Symptoms and Treatment

The term "male menopause" is used to refer to the condition of men who have hormone levels drop after mid-life.

Male menopause is a subject of controversy in the medical society. In the case of women, menopause is related with the termination of a bodily operation, like when the monthly menstruation periods stop. Also, a critical drop in the hormone levels in women occurs along with menopause. For these reasons, doctors are debating on whether male menopause really exists.

In the case of men in their middle and elderly years, smaller quantities of testosterone are being created by the testicles. This is believed to be the underlying reasons behind the occurrence of symptoms of male menopause.

Men with menopause usually suffer from irritability, sleep disturbance, low sex drive, sweating, anxiety, sadness, memory problems, and erectile dysfunction.

In most cases, erectile dysfunction may be caused by other disorders. But testosterone deficiency may be one possibility.

It is important that men who suffer from symptoms related to low levels of testosterone be subjected to medical investigations like blood tests to evaluate testosterone levels.

Other reasons for having short testosterone levels include testicular dysfunction and probable inherited features.

As a treatment, hormone replacement therapy is being recommended for men with low levels of testosterone and symptoms that come with it.

Hormone replacement may not be applicable to older men who seek treatment for their erectile dysfunction unless they actually have very minimal levels of androgen. As for younger men with known hormone deficiency, it has been proven that nominal doses of testosterone can improve interest in sex.

Testosterone replacement therapy, which is also called as androgen replacement therapy, aims to reduce the symptoms brought about by male menopause. This method is a lifelong treatment, since testosterone deficiency is generally a permanent condition.

Testosterone replacement therapy is usually given as an oral prescription, implants, or injections.

The injection of testosterone is usually carried out once every two weeks.

The oral drugs are especially prescribed to those who can't stand injections or implants.

The testosterone implants, which are being inserted under the skin of the buttock or abdomen work for a period of months. The implant works by releasing testosterone directly into the bloodstream.

Androgen therapy, however, comes with potential side effects and risks.

With low testosterone levels, the prostate tends to shrink. Hormone replacement therapy cannot recover a physically reduced prostate since it does not have influence in the levels of prostate specific antigen.

Androgen therapy may not be a cause of increased risk of prostate cancer for those who have naturally greater testosterone levels in the same age bracket.

On the other hand, the safety of hormone replacement therapy and its possible effects on the prostate, mental functioning, and cardiovascular system still need to undergo proper researches. Moreover, there is also a need to assess the probable benefits of androgen therapy on the bones and muscles.

Androgen therapy is said to increase the risk of heart diseases, although researches on this subject are uncertain. It is a known fact, however, that those with low testosterone levels have been found among heart attack victims. This opens the possibility that hormone replacement therapy could help prevent cardiovascular diseases.

Older men undiagnosed of prostate cancer should also take caution when being applied with androgens.

Sleep apnea, or the cessation of breathing during sleep, is also considered as a rare risk with hormone therapy.

Chapter 9 - What You Must Do To Treat Male Menopause

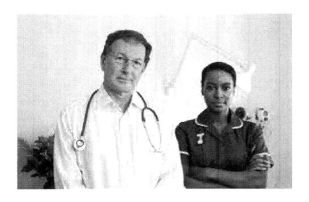

Andropause is the counterpart of menopause which is at times referred to as "male menopause." It is a type of hormonal change wherein the testosterone levels of a man depletes. It is commonly experienced by men who reaches their second adulthood, which may start as early as thirty-five or as late as sixty-five. Once a man's production of testosterone level goes down, it will bring significant change to a man's life. Depending on how a male individual will react to the situation, it may be an advantage or a disadvantage for him.

There is one fact though that will be inevitable – bothersome symptoms. For you to be able to successfully go through the "andropause stage," you need to know how to treat the said condition.

Change in lifestyle.

The food you eat, how you administer your health regime, the social activities you have and how you basically run your life is a vital factor which can contribute to the way you will respond towards male menopause.

Therefore, studies show that in order for you to combat the symptoms of andropause, you need to establish a healthy lifestyle. By doing so, you can relieve some of male menopause symptoms. By choosing the food you eat, you are most likely will be avoiding emotional exhaustion. Foods which contain too much caffeine can heighten nervousness and being nervous is one symptom which you should prevent.

Regular exercise should also be taken into account since during andropause stage sudden weight gain will be experienced. Additionally, studies show that exercise helps an individual achieve a more stable emotion.

You have to select the social activities you will be attending since it may be a factor to heighten the symptoms of male menopause. For instance, since at this stage insomnia may occur, you should do away with activities which will most likely fall on

Going Herbal

Along with establishing a healthy lifestyle, you may try herbs as a form of treatment on male menopause. There were clinical studies conducted in Europe which confirms success on andropause treatments with the use of herbs.

Helpful herbs are saw palmetto, avena sativa, eurycoma longifolia and tribulus terrestris.

Medical Treatment

Minor medical treatment includes intake of capsules and inhalation of lozenges which are common oral treatments to stabilize the testosterone level. Other male individuals have the option to go with testosterone injections since users find it effective. Another preference to even out the levels of testosterone is through the use of transdermal patches which are placed on the skin. Furthermore, a natural testosterone gel may be also be used. Some individuals who have used the gel testified to its effectiveness.

There are medical treatments appropriate for achieving the average amount of testosterone level. Testosterone replacement therapy is an alternative treatment to combat andropause wherein blood tests are being carried out to determine the amount of testosterone needed for it to normalize.

The type of treatment that you will follow depends on your personal preference and how responsible you are in undertaking the treatment option you have decided. However, it is best to discuss your desired treatment options with your physician since having too much of testosterone level is unhealthy.

If you want to overcome male menopause, you need to start with yourself. Acknowledge that you have and do what must be done to continue living the normal and happy life you once have.

Knowing the Right Treatment for Male Menopause Will Save You From the Threat of Midlife Crisis

The so called "Andropause," men hormonal change, is directly synonymous to male menopause, which leads to low testosterone level in aging men. It is said to cause depression according to Columbia University Psychiatrist, Stuart Seidman.

For several years, these changes in men's body and emotion lead them to experience a kind of midlife crisis, parallel to the experience of women in their midlife, male's version of menopause.

Majority of these men find it hard to accept that the hormones that complete their manhood are decreasing. Truth is, around 25 million of the male American population whose ages ranges from 35 to 55 are experiencing this kind of dilemma.

Hence, the Andropause, a lowering in testosterone level, is already allied to the process of normal aging for men.

If you think your age falls in the age bracket that was mentioned above, then you should take note of the possible symptoms that might have already occurred to you. The following are some of the symptoms of Andropause:

- Lowering of sex drive

- Decreasing of energy
- Lowering of strength and stamina
- Decrease of life's enjoyment
- Frequent sadness and grouchiness
- The strength of erections declined
- The sports ability is slowly deteriorating
- Falling fast asleep after taking the dinner
- Lowering of performance at work
- Repeated depression

For most medical specialists, the chief treatment for male's lowering testosterone level is the testosterone replacement therapy. Though, this treatment is presently receiving some sort of controversies because of the risks associated to its form.

In fact, doctors and their patients weigh the risks first before they venture into this kind of treatment.

On the other hand, testosterone injections also lessen the symptoms of Andropause; however, it may increase the risk of a stroke, gynecomastia or the enlargement of breasts, temporary sterility, and liver toxicity.

But don't fret; there is still another option which will not be harmful to your body. There are numerous researchers who found satisfaction in using the formulation of potent herbs for Andropause medication.

These are supplements that can be bought over the counter and will naturally increase the level of your testosterone while reducing Andropause symptoms, eliminating a large number of side effects as compared to the hormone replacement therapy.

These natural supplements will help you generate more testosterone that are originally produced in the body, thus, you will no longer need to take testosterone from the other sources, considering the fact that this only results to the slowing down of your natural testosterone production, and so, putting you in a bad situation after you cease taking the injections.

Therefore, it is more preferable that you take this kind of treatment than having medications that could be harmful to your body.

If you are planning to purchase this herbal supplements, it is advisable that before buying try to analyze first the products. Make sure that includes the following: the potential to augment physical performance, endurance, and stamina, while maintaining the heightened intensity of testosterone as well as the energy.

Look for the list that represents the finest products that are offered for the consumer. Choose the products which will present the most efficient formulas with the supreme potential to bring utmost performance.

Male Menopause: How Treatments Work

Menopause is what women experience when they reach a certain age where their bodies stop producing hormones. It is a point where women will no longer be able to reproduce and it is also a point where their lives will change.

However, it is also a fact that males also experience this kind of condition. It has been found that men will also experience the so-called male menopause when they reach a certain age. But unlike women where they stop producing hormones instantly, men experience a decline in production of hormones.

Sometimes, male menopause is also called the mid-life crisis where male hormone levels drop that often results to depression, anxiety, and decline of interest in sex. As a male, you have to prepare to face this condition because when you reach a certain age (usually at late 50's to early 60's); you will also experience this condition.

First of all, you need to be able to identify the signs and symptoms of male menopause. Usually, the symptoms are very much like what a female experiences when they go through menopause. It will include depression, irritability, sadness, low interest in sex, anxiety, hot flashes, sweating, erectile dysfunction, concentration problems, and memory problems.

Erectile dysfunction can also be caused by other conditions, such as a disease. However, the low testosterone level can also contribute to this condition.

If you suspect that you are going through male menopause, it is recommended that you should consult your doctor about it first before jumping into a conclusion and getting treated for it. The doctor will conduct a series of tests to confirm that you are really going through male menopause. To do this, the doctor will test your testosterone level and also your symptoms. If it is indeed male menopause, the doctor can recommend treatments to ease the symptoms.

Today, there are already treatments for male menopause where it can make it easier for you to cope up with the condition. It will not necessarily mean that it can treat the condition, but you have to consider that the treatment's aim for male menopause, like female menopause, is to lessen the symptoms.

There is hormone replacement therapy for men who have low testosterone level. This treatment can help you lessen the symptoms associated with male menopause. This treatment is called testosterone replacement therapy. With this treatment, you can lessen the effects of male menopause and can definitely help you go through it.

In fact, this therapy has been found effective. It gradually increased the muscle mass, the mental functioning, bone density and it also enabled men to get interested in sex again.

However, testosterone replacement therapy should only be done with close supervision of a professional. Too much of testosterone injected in your body can produce unwanted side effects. The professional will be able to adjust the doses in accordance with the effects you experience during your first testosterone replacement therapy.

In time and also after a few sessions, the professional will be able to know the correct dosage for you.

If you cannot tolerate the injections, there are also oral capsules that you can take for this therapy. There are also testosterone patches where it can provide a steady release of testosterone.

If you don't want this therapy through injection, through oral capsules, or through patches, you can consider getting implants. The testosterone implants are inserted in the lower abdomen or hip under anesthetic. This can provide treatment that can last up to 6 months.

These are the treatments that you can consider when you are going through male menopause. So, if you are at that certain age where sex doesn't interest you anymore, and where you are more motherly, you can consider getting a testosterone replacement therapy. Always remember that this therapy should only be done with close supervision of a professional to avoid unwanted side effects.

I Have a Special Gift for My Readers

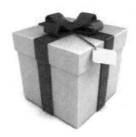

I appreciate my readers for without them I am just another struggling author attempting to make ends meet.

My readers and I have in common a passion for the written word as well as the desire to learn and grow from books.

My special offer to you is a massive ebook library that I have compiled over the years. It contains hundreds of fiction and non-fiction ebooks in Adobe Acrobat PDF format as well as the Greek classics and old literary classics too.

In fact, this library is so massive to completely download the entire library will require over 5 GBs open on your desktop.

Use the link below and scan all of the ebooks in the library. You can select the ebooks you want individually or download the entire library.

The link below does not expire after a given time period so you are free to return for more books rather than clog your desktop. And feel free to give the link to your friends who enjoy reading too.

I thank you for reading my book and hope if you are pleased that you will leave me an honest review so that I can improve my work and or write books that appeal to your interests.

Okay, here is the link...

http://tinyurl.com/special-readers-promo

PS: If you wish to reach me personally for any reason you may simply write to mailto:support@epubwealth.com.

I answer all of my emails so rest assured I will respond.

Meet the Author
Dr. Treat Preston is a behavioral scientist specializing in all types of relationships and associated problems, psychological triggers as applied to commercial advertising and marketing, and energy psychology. He is a best-selling author with numerous books dealing on publishing, behavioral science, marketing and more. He is also one of the lead research scientists with AppliedMindSciences.com, the mind research unit of ForensicsNation.com.

He and his wife Cynthia reside in Auburn, California.

Visit some of his websites
http://www.AddMeInNow.com
http://www.AppliedMindSciences.com
http://www.AppliedWebInfo.com
http://www.BookbuilderPLUS.com
http://www.BookJumping.com
http://www.EmailNations.com
http://www.EmbarrassingProblemsFix.com
http://www.ePubWealth.com
http://www.ForensicsNation.com
http://www.ForensicsNationStore.com
http://www.FreebiesNation.com
http://www.HealthFitnessWellnessNation.com
http://www.Neternatives.com
http://www.PrivacyNations.com
http://www.RetireWithoutMoney.org
http://www.SurvivalNations.com
http://www.TheBentonKitchen.com
http://www.Theolegions.org
http://www.VideoBookbuilder.com

Printed in Great Britain
by Amazon